1.

You always...

2.

You are the first to...

3.

You love...

4.

You help...

5.

You choose...

6.

You challenge...

7.

You don't worry about...

8.

You accept...

9.

You appreciate...

10.

You encourage...

11.

You are an incredible...

12.

You give...

13.

You answer...

14.

You are the least...

15.

You never...

16.

You have a...

17.

You think...

18.

You hate...

19.

You love to...

20.

You aren't afraid to...

21.

You are
an amazing...

22.

You understand...

23.

You remember...

24.

Every day you...

25.

You believe...

26.

You inspire...

27.

You make...

28.

You have a wonderful...

29.

You celebrate...

30.

You are
the most...

31.

You have...

32.

You are...

Made in the USA
Coppell, TX
09 June 2020

27173656R10046